Slimming Smoothies: Tasty Recipes for Rapid Weight Loss

Healthy Eating

Table of contents

Introduction

Welcome to Slimming Smoothies: Tasty Recipes for Rapid Weight Loss. In the quest for better health and fitness, it's no secret that what we consume plays a pivotal role. Smoothies, with their delicious blend of flavors, offer a delightful way to nourish your body while working towards your weight loss goals. In this book, we present a collection of mouthwatering smoothie recipes carefully crafted to help you on your journey to a healthier, slimmer you. Smoothies have gained immense popularity in recent years for several compelling reasons. They are not just refreshing beverages; they are nutritional powerhouses packed with vitamins, minerals, fiber, and antioxidants. When prepared with the right ingredients, smoothies can be an effective tool for weight loss and overall well-being.

Why Smoothies for Weight Loss?

Before diving into the delicious recipes, it's essential to understand why smoothies can be a valuable addition to your weight loss plan:

1. Nutrient Density: Smoothies allow you to pack a variety of nutrient-dense foods into one convenient glass. By blending fruits, vegetables, nuts, seeds, and other wholesome ingredients, you create a nutrient-rich concoction that can keep you feeling full and satisfied.

2. Portion Control: One of the challenges in weight management is controlling portion sizes. Smoothies offer portion control naturally. Each recipe provides a measured serving, making it easier to manage your calorie intake.

3. Satiety: The combination of fiber, protein, and healthy fats in many smoothies can help keep hunger at bay, reducing the urge to snack on less healthy options throughout the day.

4. Customization: Smoothies are incredibly versatile. You can tailor them to your taste preferences and dietary needs. Whether you're vegan, gluten-free, or following a specific diet plan, there's a smoothie recipe here for you.

5. Hydration: Staying hydrated is essential for overall health and can support weight loss. Many smoothie ingredients, like fruits and vegetables, have high water content, helping you meet your daily hydration goals.

6. Convenience: In our busy lives, convenience matters. Smoothies are quick to prepare and can be enjoyed on the go. They are an excellent choice for a healthy breakfast, post-workout snack, or anytime you need a nutritious boost.

7. Flavor Variety: Variety is key to a sustainable weight loss journey. With several unique recipes to choose from, you won't get bored, and you'll discover exciting new flavors that make healthy eating enjoyable.

Creating Your Weight Loss Success
Successful weight loss isn't about deprivation or following extreme diets. It's about making sustainable, positive changes to your eating habits. Smoothies can be a part of that equation,

5. Dietary Modifications: We understand that dietary restrictions and preferences vary. For each recipe, we offer suggestions for modifications to accommodate various diets, including vegetarian, vegan, gluten-free, and low-sugar options.

6. Beautiful Imagery: Visual appeal can be a significant motivator. You'll find vibrant, high-quality images of each smoothie to inspire your culinary creations.

7. Shopping Lists: To simplify your smoothie-making journey, we've included comprehensive shopping lists at the beginning of each category chapter. These lists outline the ingredients you'll need to create the recipes within that section.

Embarking on a journey towards weight loss and improved health is a commendable decision. It's important to remember that this journey is unique to you, and it should be enjoyable and sustainable. These smoothie recipes are designed to support your goals while indulging your taste buds.

Incorporate these smoothies into your daily routine, experiment with different flavors, and find your favorites. Alongside a balanced diet and regular physical activity, these smoothies can be a valuable tool in your quest for a healthier, happier you.

Now, let's begin this exciting journey through the world of Slimming Smoothies. Whether you're looking for a morning energy boost, a post-workout recovery drink, or a guilt-free dessert, you'll find it within these pages. Cheers to your health, your well-being, and the delicious path ahead!

Green Goddess Detox Smoothie

The Green Goddess Detox Smoothie is a vibrant, nutrient-packed concoction that's perfect for jump-starting your day or cleansing your body after indulgent moments. Packed with an array of green ingredients, this smoothie provides a natural detoxifying effect while delivering a burst of essential vitamins and minerals. It's a refreshing and revitalizing choice for those looking to boost their energy levels and support their body's detoxification processes.

Ingredients:

- 1 cup of fresh spinach leaves
- 1/2 cucumber, peeled and sliced
- 1/2 green apple, cored and chopped
- 1/2 lemon, juiced
- 1 small piece of fresh ginger (about 1 inch), peeled
- 1 tablespoon of chia seeds

- 1/2 cup of unsweetened almond milk (or your preferred milk)
- Ice cubes (optional)

Nutritional Benefits:

The Green Goddess Detox Smoothie is a nutrient powerhouse that offers several health benefits:

- Leafy Greens: Spinach provides a rich source of vitamins A and K, along with essential minerals like iron and calcium. It's also a great source of fiber, which aids digestion.

- Cucumber: Cucumber is known for its hydrating properties and is low in calories. It contributes to the smoothie's refreshing nature.

- Green Apple: Green apples add a touch of natural sweetness while providing vitamins C and fiber.

- Lemon: Lemon juice adds zesty flavor and offers vitamin C, known for its immune-boosting properties.

- Ginger: Ginger adds a spicy kick and is renowned for its potential anti-inflammatory and digestion-aiding properties.

- Chia Seeds: Chia seeds are packed with fiber, protein, and healthy fats. They also absorb liquid, helping to thicken the smoothie and keep you feeling full.

- Almond Milk: Unsweetened almond milk is a low-calorie dairy alternative that complements the flavors of the smoothie without adding unnecessary sugars.

Instructions:

1. Start by adding the fresh spinach leaves to your blender. Spinach is not only incredibly nutritious but also blends well, providing a smooth texture to your smoothie.

2. Follow with the cucumber slices and chopped green apple. These ingredients contribute to the smoothie's refreshing taste and add a natural sweetness.

3. Squeeze the juice of half a lemon into the blender. The lemon juice not only enhances the flavor but also provides a burst of vitamin C.

4. Grate or finely chop the fresh ginger (about 1 inch in size) and add it to the mix. Ginger adds a delightful zing and offers potential digestive benefits.

5. To boost the nutritional value of your smoothie and add a dose of healthy omega-3 fatty acids, sprinkle in a tablespoon of chia seeds.

6. Pour in your choice of unsweetened almond milk (or preferred milk). Adjust the quantity to achieve your desired smoothie thickness.

7. If you prefer a colder smoothie, feel free to toss in a handful of ice cubes.

8. Blend all the ingredients until you achieve a smooth, creamy consistency.

9. Taste your Green Goddess Detox Smoothie and adjust the flavor to your liking. You can add a bit more lemon juice for tanginess or a touch of honey or maple syrup for extra sweetness if desired.

Serving Suggestion
Pour your freshly blended Green Goddess Detox Smoothie into a chilled glass. Garnish with a thin cucumber slice or a sprinkle of chia seeds for an added visual appeal. This smoothie is best enjoyed immediately to savor its fresh, invigorating flavors fully.

Berry Blast Breakfast Smoothie

The Berry Blast Breakfast Smoothie is your ticket to a vibrant, delicious, and energy-packed morning. Bursting with the natural sweetness and antioxidant-rich goodness of mixed berries, this smoothie is designed to kickstart your day on a healthy note. It's a delightful way to satisfy your morning hunger while providing a substantial dose of vitamins and fiber.

Ingredients:

- 1/2 cup of frozen mixed berries (strawberries, blueberries, raspberries, and blackberries)
- 1/2 banana (frozen or fresh)
- 1/2 cup of Greek yogurt (or a dairy-free alternative)
- 1 tablespoon of honey (optional for added sweetness)
- 1/2 cup of unsweetened almond milk (or your preferred milk)

- 1 tablespoon of rolled oats (for added fiber and thickness)
- A handful of ice cubes (optional)

Nutritional Benefits:

The Berry Blast Breakfast Smoothie is not just a tasty treat; it's also loaded with health benefits:

- Mixed Berries: Berries are packed with antioxidants, vitamins, and fiber. They can help boost your immune system, support heart health, and improve digestion.

- Banana: Banana adds natural sweetness and creaminess to the smoothie. It's a great source of potassium, which can help regulate blood pressure and maintain proper muscle function.

- Greek Yogurt: Greek yogurt provides a creamy texture and a protein boost. It's rich in probiotics, which promote gut health and aid digestion.

- Honey (Optional): Honey can add sweetness if desired, and it may offer potential antibacterial and anti-inflammatory properties.

- Almond Milk: Unsweetened almond milk is a low-calorie dairy alternative that complements the flavors without adding unnecessary sugars.

- Rolled Oats: Oats provide fiber, which can help keep you feeling full and satisfied throughout the morning.

Instructions:

1. Start by placing the frozen mixed berries into your blender. The frozen berries will give your smoothie a refreshing, icy consistency.

2. Add the banana to the blender. If you prefer a thicker smoothie, consider using a frozen banana. This will also enhance the creaminess.

3. Spoon in the Greek yogurt. Greek yogurt adds creaminess and a protein boost to your smoothie.

4. If you desire extra sweetness, add a tablespoon of honey. Adjust the amount to your taste preference.

5. Pour in your choice of unsweetened almond milk (or your preferred milk) to create the desired consistency. The quantity can be adjusted to your liking.

6. To add fiber and thickness to your smoothie, toss in a tablespoon of rolled oats.

7. If you prefer a colder, more chilled smoothie, consider adding a handful of ice cubes.

8. Blend all the ingredients until you achieve a smooth, luscious texture. The color should be a beautiful, vibrant shade of purple.

9. Taste your Berry Blast Breakfast Smoothie and adjust the flavor if necessary. You can add more honey for sweetness or more almond milk for a thinner consistency.

Serving Suggestion:
Pour your freshly blended Berry Blast Breakfast Smoothie into a tall glass. Garnish with a few fresh berries or a banana slice to enhance the presentation. This smoothie is best enjoyed in the morning to kickstart your day with a burst of energy and flavor.

The Berry Blast Breakfast Smoothie is not only a treat for your taste buds but also a nutritious powerhouse to fuel your morning. Its mix of vibrant berries, creamy yogurt, and natural sweetness from banana and honey creates a delightful balance of flavors. Make this smoothie a part of your breakfast routine to ensure you're starting your day with a boost of antioxidants, fiber, and essential nutrients. It's a delicious way to nourish your body while enjoying the convenience of a quick and satisfying morning meal.

Tropical Paradise Protein Smoothie

Imagine sipping on a taste of the tropics right at your breakfast table. The Tropical Paradise Protein Smoothie is a refreshing and protein-packed creation designed to transport you to an island getaway with each sip. This smoothie combines the vibrant flavors of tropical fruits with the power of protein to kickstart your day on a healthy and energizing note.

Ingredients:

- 1/2 cup of frozen mango chunks
- 1/2 cup of frozen pineapple chunks
- 1/2 banana (frozen or fresh)
- 1/2 cup of Greek yogurt (or a dairy-free alternative)
- 1 scoop of vanilla protein powder (your choice of plant-based or whey)
- 1 tablespoon of shredded coconut (optional, for added tropical flair)

- 1/2 cup of coconut milk (or your preferred milk)
- A handful of ice cubes (optional)

Nutritional Benefits:

The Tropical Paradise Protein Smoothie is more than just a vacation for your taste buds. It's a nutritional powerhouse:

- Mango: Mango is rich in vitamins A and C, providing immune-boosting benefits and promoting healthy skin.

- Pineapple: Pineapple is loaded with vitamin C and the enzyme bromelain, which can aid digestion.

- Banana: Banana adds creaminess and natural sweetness, along with potassium to support muscle function.

- Greek Yogurt: Greek yogurt adds creaminess and a protein boost to keep you feeling full and satisfied.

- Protein Powder: Protein powder is essential for muscle repair and growth, making it a valuable addition to your morning routine.

- Shredded Coconut (Optional): Shredded coconut contributes a delightful tropical flavor and a touch of healthy fats.

- Coconut Milk: Coconut milk enhances the tropical theme and complements the flavors without adding unnecessary sugars.

Instructions:

1. Start by adding the frozen mango chunks to your blender. The frozen mango lends a creamy texture and that tropical sweetness.

2. Follow with the frozen or fresh banana. A frozen banana will enhance creaminess.

3. Add the frozen pineapple chunks for that unmistakable tropical tang.

4. Spoon in the Greek yogurt, which not only adds creaminess but also provides a protein punch.

5. Include a scoop of vanilla protein powder of your choice (plant-based or whey) to boost your protein intake.

6. If you desire an extra touch of tropical flair, add a tablespoon of shredded coconut.

7. Pour in your choice of coconut milk (or your preferred milk) to create the desired consistency. Adjust the quantity to your liking.

8. For an even colder and frostier experience, consider adding a handful of ice cubes.

9. Blend all the ingredients until you achieve a smooth, velvety texture. The color should resemble a sunny day in paradise.

10. Taste your Tropical Paradise Protein Smoothie and adjust the flavor if necessary. You can add more coconut milk for creaminess or more protein powder for an extra protein boost.

Serving Suggestion:
Pour your freshly blended Tropical Paradise Protein Smoothie into a tropical-themed glass. Garnish with a sprinkle of shredded coconut and a small slice of pineapple or a mango cube for that authentic tropical touch. This smoothie is a delightful way to infuse your morning routine with the flavors of a tropical getaway.

The Tropical Paradise Protein Smoothie is your daily ticket to an island escape, right in your kitchen. It offers a delightful balance of tropical flavors, creaminess, and protein power to fuel your day. Make this smoothie a part of your morning ritual, and you'll feel refreshed, nourished, and ready to conquer whatever the day brings. It's a flavorful reminder that eating healthily can be an exciting and tasty adventure, even if you're miles away from the nearest beach.

Spinach and Pineapple Slimdown Smoothie:

If you're on a mission to shed pounds and boost your energy levels, the Spinach and Pineapple Slimdown Smoothie is your ally in this journey. This vibrant green smoothie combines the leafy goodness of spinach with the tropical sweetness of pineapple to create a refreshing and revitalizing blend that supports your weight loss goals.

Ingredients:
- 1 cup of fresh spinach leaves
- 1 cup of frozen pineapple chunks
- 1/2 banana (frozen or fresh)
- 1/2 cup of Greek yogurt (or a dairy-free alternative)
- 1 tablespoon of honey (optional, for added sweetness)
- 1/2 cup of coconut water (or your preferred liquid)
- A handful of ice cubes (optional)

Nutritional Benefits:
The Spinach and Pineapple Slimdown Smoothie
is a nutrient-packed powerhouse:

- Spinach: Spinach is rich in vitamins A and K,
iron, and fiber. It supports digestion and
provides essential nutrients without adding many
calories.

- Pineapple: Pineapple contributes natural
sweetness, vitamin C, and bromelain, an enzyme
that aids digestion.

- Banana: Banana adds creaminess and
potassium, which is essential for muscle
function and maintaining proper blood pressure.

- Greek Yogurt: Greek yogurt adds creaminess
and a protein boost, helping you feel full and
satisfied.

- Honey (Optional): Honey can enhance sweetness if desired and may offer potential antibacterial and anti-inflammatory benefits.

- Coconut Water: Coconut water provides hydration and complements the tropical theme without added sugars.

Instructions:
1. Begin by placing the fresh spinach leaves into your blender. Spinach blends well and provides a beautiful green color.

2. Add the frozen pineapple chunks to the blender. The frozen pineapple will give your smoothie a refreshing, icy texture.

3. Include the frozen or fresh banana for natural sweetness and creaminess.

4. Spoon in the Greek yogurt to add creaminess and a protein boost.

5. If you desire extra sweetness, add a tablespoon of honey. Adjust the amount based on your taste preference.

6. Pour in your choice of coconut water (or your preferred liquid) to create the desired consistency. You can adjust the quantity to achieve your preferred thickness.

7. If you prefer a colder, frostier smoothie, consider adding a handful of ice cubes.

8. Blend all the ingredients until you achieve a smooth, velvety texture. The result should be a vibrant green color that's both appealing and nutritious.

9. Taste your Spinach and Pineapple Slimdown Smoothie and adjust the flavor to your liking. You can add more honey for sweetness or more coconut water for a thinner consistency.
Serving Suggestion:
Pour your freshly blended Spinach and
Pineapple Slimdown Smoothie into a tall glass.

Garnish with a pineapple slice or a sprig of fresh mint to add a touch of elegance. This smoothie is best enjoyed as a revitalizing breakfast option or a mid-day pick-me-up, helping you stay on track with your weight loss goals.

The Spinach and Pineapple Slimdown Smoothie is a green powerhouse that makes healthy eating a delightful experience. Its blend of spinach, pineapple, and creamy yogurt creates a balanced and refreshing flavor profile. Incorporate this smoothie into your daily routine to enjoy the benefits of essential nutrients while working towards your weight loss objectives. It's a delicious reminder that taking care of your body can be as enjoyable as it is beneficial.

Peanut Butter Banana Bliss

The Peanut Butter Banana Bliss smoothie is a taste of pure indulgence without the guilt. If you're looking for a creamy, protein-packed treat that can satisfy your sweet tooth while supporting your weight loss journey, look no further. This delightful blend combines the rich, nutty flavor of peanut butter with the natural sweetness of bananas for a truly blissful experience.

Ingredients:

- 2 ripe bananas (frozen or fresh)
- 2 tablespoons of natural peanut butter (no added sugar or salt)
- 1/2 cup of Greek yogurt (or a dairy-free alternative)
- 1 tablespoon of honey (optional, for added sweetness)
- 1/2 cup of unsweetened almond milk (or your preferred milk)

- A handful of ice cubes (optional)

Nutritional Benefits:

The Peanut Butter Banana Bliss smoothie offers more than just heavenly flavor; it's also a nutritional powerhouse:

- Bananas: Bananas provide natural sweetness and a good dose of potassium, which supports muscle function and overall health.

- Natural Peanut Butter: Peanut butter adds rich, nutty flavor and healthy fats, along with protein to keep you feeling full.

- Greek Yogurt: Greek yogurt contributes creaminess and additional protein, promoting satiety.

- Honey (Optional): Honey can enhance sweetness if desired, and it offers potential antibacterial and anti-inflammatory properties.

- Almond Milk: Unsweetened almond milk complements the flavors without adding unnecessary sugars.

Instructions:

1. Begin by peeling and slicing the ripe bananas. If you prefer a thicker, creamier texture, use frozen bananas.

2. Add the banana slices to your blender. The natural sweetness of bananas will be the foundation of your blissful smoothie.

3. Spoon in two tablespoons of natural peanut butter. Be sure to select one without added sugar or salt for a healthier option.

4. Include the Greek yogurt for creaminess and an extra protein boost.

5. If you desire added sweetness, add a tablespoon of honey. Adjust the amount based on your taste preference.

6. Pour in your choice of unsweetened almond milk (or your preferred milk) to create the desired consistency. Adjust the quantity to achieve your preferred thickness.

7. If you prefer an icier, frostier smoothie, consider adding a handful of ice cubes.

8. Blend all the ingredients until you achieve a smooth, velvety texture. The result should be a luscious, creamy blend of banana and peanut butter flavors.

9. Taste your Peanut Butter Banana Bliss smoothie and adjust the flavor if necessary. You can add more honey for sweetness or more almond milk for a thinner consistency.

Serving Suggestion:

Pour your freshly blended Peanut Butter Banana Bliss into a chilled glass. Garnish with a drizzle of peanut butter or a banana slice for a touch of elegance. This smoothie is ideal for breakfast or as a satisfying post-workout recovery drink. It's a delicious reminder that healthy choices can be downright blissful.:

The Peanut Butter Banana Bliss smoothie is a delightful balance of indulgence and nutrition. Its rich and creamy combination of peanut butter and banana creates a satisfying treat that's perfect for those moments when you're craving something sweet but don't want to derail your weight loss goals. Enjoy this smoothie as a guilt-free pleasure that nourishes both your taste buds and your body, reminding you that healthy eating can indeed be blissful.

Blueberry Almond Delight

The Blueberry Almond Delight smoothie is a delightful blend of flavors that marries the sweet and tangy allure of blueberries with the nutty richness of almonds. This smoothie is not only a treat for your taste buds but also a nutritional powerhouse. Loaded with antioxidants and healthy fats, it's the perfect choice for those looking to enjoy a guilt-free, satisfying snack or meal replacement.

Ingredients:
- 1 cup of fresh or frozen blueberries
- 1/4 cup of raw almonds
- 1/2 banana (frozen or fresh)
- 1/2 cup of Greek yogurt (or a dairy-free alternative)
- 1 tablespoon of honey (optional, for added sweetness)
- 1/2 cup of unsweetened almond milk (or your preferred milk)
- A handful of ice cubes (optional)

Nutritional Benefits:
The Blueberry Almond Delight smoothie offers
an array of health benefits:

- Blueberries: Blueberries are renowned for their
high antioxidant content, which supports cellular
health and may aid in weight management.

- Raw Almonds: Almonds are packed with
healthy fats, fiber, and protein, which promote
feelings of fullness and satisfaction.

- Banana: Banana contributes natural sweetness,
creaminess, and potassium, an essential mineral
for overall health.

- Greek Yogurt: Greek yogurt adds creaminess
and an additional protein boost, aiding in satiety.

- Honey (Optional): Honey can enhance
sweetness if desired, and it offers potential
antibacterial and anti-inflammatory properties.

- Almond Milk: Unsweetened almond milk
complements the flavors without adding
unnecessary sugars.

Instructions:
1. Start by adding the blueberries to your
blender. Whether fresh or frozen, blueberries
lend a vibrant color and a burst of antioxidants.

2. Add the raw almonds for their nutty richness
and the heart-healthy fats they bring to the mix.

3. Include the banana, which adds natural
sweetness and creaminess to the smoothie.

4. Spoon in the Greek yogurt for its creaminess
and an extra boost of protein.

5. If you desire extra sweetness, add a
tablespoon of honey. Adjust the amount based
on your taste preference.

6. Pour in your choice of unsweetened almond
milk (or your preferred milk) to create the

desired consistency. You can adjust the quantity to achieve your preferred thickness.

7. If you prefer a colder, frostier smoothie, consider adding a handful of ice cubes.

8. Blend all the ingredients until you achieve a smooth, velvety texture. The result should be a luscious blend of blueberry and almond flavors.

9. Taste your Blueberry Almond Delight smoothie and adjust the flavor if necessary. You can add more honey for sweetness or more almond milk for a thinner consistency.

Serving Suggestion:

Pour your freshly blended Blueberry Almond Delight smoothie into a chilled glass. Garnish with a few fresh blueberries or a sprinkle of crushed almonds for an extra visual and textural dimension. This smoothie is perfect for breakfast, as a mid-day pick-me-up, or as a post-workout refueling option. It's a reminder that

delicious and healthy can coexist in perfect
harmony.

The Blueberry Almond Delight smoothie is a
testament to the idea that nutritious choices can
be both delicious and satisfying. Its blend of
blueberries and almonds provides a unique
combination of flavors and textures that will
tantalize your taste buds while nourishing your
body with essential nutrients. Make this
smoothie a regular part of your routine to enjoy
the benefits of antioxidants, healthy fats, and
protein without sacrificing indulgence. It's a
delightful reminder that the path to wellness can
be both enjoyable and nutritious.

Kale and Mango Magic

The Kale and Mango Magic smoothie is a nutritional powerhouse that brings together the earthy goodness of kale and the tropical sweetness of mango. This dynamic combination creates a refreshing and revitalizing blend that's not only delicious but also incredibly beneficial for your health. If you're looking for a green smoothie that packs a punch in flavor and nutrients, this one's a true magic trick.

Ingredients:

- 1 cup of fresh kale leaves, stems removed
- 1 cup of ripe mango chunks (fresh or frozen)
- 1/2 banana (frozen or fresh)
- 1/2 cup of Greek yogurt (or a dairy-free alternative)
- 1 tablespoon of honey (optional, for added sweetness)
- 1/2 cup of coconut water (or your preferred liquid)

- A handful of ice cubes (optional)

Nutritional Benefits:

The Kale and Mango Magic smoothie offers a wide array of health benefits:

- Kale: Kale is a nutritional powerhouse, rich in vitamins A, C, and K, along with essential minerals and fiber.

- Mango: Mango provides natural sweetness, vitamin C, and dietary fiber to support digestion.

- Banana: Banana adds creaminess, natural sweetness, and potassium for overall health.

- Greek Yogurt: Greek yogurt contributes creaminess and an additional protein boost to promote satiety.

- Honey (Optional): Honey can enhance sweetness if desired, and it offers potential antibacterial and anti-inflammatory properties.

- Coconut Water: Coconut water complements the tropical theme and provides hydration without added sugars.

Instructions:

1. Start by adding the fresh kale leaves to your blender. Kale is known for its incredible nutrient density and vibrant green color.

2. Follow with the ripe mango chunks, whether fresh or frozen. The mango's natural sweetness will be a highlight of your smoothie.

3. Add the frozen or fresh banana for extra creaminess and sweetness.

4. Spoon in the Greek yogurt to add creaminess and an extra protein boost.

5. If you desire added sweetness, add a tablespoon of honey. Adjust the amount based on your taste preference.

6. Pour in your choice of coconut water (or your preferred liquid) to create the desired consistency. Adjust the quantity to achieve your preferred thickness.

7. If you prefer a colder, frostier smoothie, consider adding a handful of ice cubes.

8. Blend all the ingredients until you achieve a smooth, vibrant green texture that resembles liquid magic.

9. Taste your Kale and Mango Magic smoothie and adjust the flavor if necessary. You can add more honey for sweetness or more coconut water for a thinner consistency.

Serving Suggestion:

Pour your freshly blended Kale and Mango Magic smoothie into a tall glass. Garnish with a slice of fresh mango or a kale leaf for an extra touch of freshness. This smoothie is ideal for breakfast, as a post-workout recovery option, or simply as a way to infuse your day with the vibrant flavors of kale and mango.

The Kale and Mango Magic smoothie is a delightful reminder that green can be both delicious and nutritious. Its blend of kale's earthy depth and mango's tropical sweetness creates a harmonious flavor profile that's as vibrant as its appearance. Incorporate this smoothie into your routine to enjoy the benefits of essential nutrients and antioxidants while savoring the magic of a well-balanced and refreshing drink. It's a testament to how healthy choices can be both satisfying and enchanting.

Chocolate Protein Powerhouse

Indulgence meets nutrition in the Chocolate Protein Powerhouse smoothie. If you're seeking a guilt-free treat that satisfies your chocolate cravings while providing a substantial protein boost, this smoothie is your answer. It combines the rich, velvety flavor of chocolate with the power of protein for a delightful and nourishing experience.

Ingredients:

- 1 ripe banana (frozen or fresh)
- 1 scoop of chocolate protein powder (your choice of plant-based or whey)
- 2 tablespoons of natural unsweetened cocoa powder
- 1/2 cup of Greek yogurt (or a dairy-free alternative)
- 1 tablespoon of almond butter (or your preferred nut butter)

- 1 tablespoon of honey (optional, for added sweetness)
- 1/2 cup of unsweetened almond milk (or your preferred milk)
- A handful of ice cubes (optional)

Nutritional Benefits:

The Chocolate Protein Powerhouse smoothie offers a delightful blend of flavors and a variety of health benefits:

- Banana: Banana adds creaminess, natural sweetness, and potassium for overall health.

- Chocolate Protein Powder: Chocolate protein powder infuses the smoothie with rich flavor and helps with muscle recovery and growth.

- Cocoa Powder: Unsweetened cocoa powder provides chocolatey goodness without added sugar and offers antioxidants.

- Greek Yogurt: Greek yogurt contributes creaminess and an extra protein boost to promote satiety.

- Almond Butter: Almond butter adds nutty richness and healthy fats for satiety.

- Honey (Optional): Honey can enhance sweetness if desired, and it offers potential antibacterial and anti-inflammatory properties.

- Almond Milk: Unsweetened almond milk complements the flavors without adding unnecessary sugars.

Instructions:

1. Start by peeling and slicing the ripe banana. If you prefer a thicker, creamier texture, use a frozen banana.

2. Add the banana slices to your blender. The natural sweetness of bananas serves as the foundation of your chocolate delight.

3. Include a scoop of chocolate protein powder of your choice (plant-based or whey) for a protein-packed punch and rich chocolate flavor.

4. Spoon in the unsweetened cocoa powder to intensify the chocolate goodness without adding sugar.

5. Add the Greek yogurt to create creaminess and increase the protein content.

6. Include a tablespoon of almond butter (or your preferred nut butter) to add nutty richness and healthy fats.

7. If you desire added sweetness, add a tablespoon of honey. Adjust the amount based on your taste preference.

8. Pour in your choice of unsweetened almond milk (or your preferred milk) to create the desired consistency. You can adjust the quantity to achieve your preferred thickness.

but it's crucial to remember that they are not a magic solution. They work best when integrated into a balanced diet and an active lifestyle.

In this book, we've curated a wide range of smoothie recipes to cater to different tastes and dietary preferences. Whether you're a fan of tropical fruits, leafy greens, or rich chocolates, there's a smoothie for you. Each recipe is designed with weight loss in mind, using ingredients that support your goals while satisfying your taste buds.

Navigating the Book
Before we dive into the recipes, let's take a moment to explore how this book is organized and how you can make the most of it:
1. Nutritional Information: We understand the importance of transparency in your weight loss journey. For each smoothie recipe, we provide detailed nutritional information, including calories, macronutrients (carbohydrates, protein, fat), fiber content, and essential vitamins and minerals. This information empowers you to

make informed choices and track your progress effectively.

2. Ingredient Profiles: In addition to nutritional information, we provide insights into the key ingredients used in each smoothie. Learn about the health benefits of ingredients like kale, chia seeds, berries, and more. Understanding the nutritional value of these ingredients can help you make smarter choices in your overall diet.

3. Serving Suggestions: While smoothies are delightful on their own, we also offer serving suggestions and creative toppings to enhance your smoothie experience. These tips can elevate your enjoyment and make each smoothie a satisfying meal or snack.

4. Tips and Tricks: Throughout the book, you'll find helpful tips and tricks to make the smoothie-making process even more enjoyable and efficient. From freezing fruits for a thicker texture to using the right blender settings, these insights will prove invaluable.

9. If you prefer a colder, more refreshing smoothie, consider adding a handful of ice cubes.

10. Blend all the ingredients until you achieve a smooth, velvety texture. The result should be a rich, chocolatey delight.

11. Taste your Chocolate Protein Powerhouse smoothie and adjust the flavor if necessary. You can add more honey for sweetness or more almond milk for a thinner consistency.

Serving Suggestion:

Pour your freshly blended Chocolate Protein Powerhouse smoothie into a chilled glass. For an extra touch of chocolate elegance, garnish with a sprinkle of cocoa powder or a drizzle of melted dark chocolate. This smoothie is perfect for breakfast, as a post-workout recovery option, or as a healthier way to satisfy your chocolate cravings. It's a reminder that nutritious choices can be both decadent and energizing.

Cucumber Mint Cooler

When it comes to revitalizing and hydrating, the Cucumber Mint Cooler smoothie is a true champion. This refreshing blend combines the crispness of cucumber with the invigorating essence of mint, resulting in a delightful beverage that not only quenches your thirst but also provides a dose of essential vitamins and minerals. It's the perfect choice for a hot summer day or any time you need a revitalizing pick-me-up.

Ingredients:

- 1 cucumber, peeled and sliced
- A handful of fresh mint leaves
- Juice of 1 lime
- 1 tablespoon of honey (optional, for added sweetness)
- 1/2 cup of Greek yogurt (or a dairy-free alternative)

- 1/2 cup of coconut water (or your preferred liquid)
- Ice cubes (optional)

Nutritional Benefits:

The Cucumber Mint Cooler smoothie is not just about refreshment; it also offers several health benefits:

- Cucumber: Cucumber is known for its high water content, making it an excellent choice for hydration. It also provides vitamins and minerals, including vitamin K and potassium.

- Mint: Mint leaves lend a refreshing and invigorating flavor while potentially aiding digestion.

- Lime: Lime juice adds zesty citrus flavor and provides a burst of vitamin C, known for its immune-boosting properties.

- Honey (Optional): Honey can enhance sweetness if desired and may offer potential antibacterial and anti-inflammatory benefits.

- Greek Yogurt: Greek yogurt adds creaminess and a dose of protein, promoting satiety.

- Coconut Water: Coconut water complements the flavors and offers hydration without added sugars.

Instructions:

1. Begin by peeling and slicing the cucumber. Removing the peel helps create a smoother texture.

2. Add the sliced cucumber to your blender. Cucumber's high water content is the base for your cooling smoothie.

3. Toss in a handful of fresh mint leaves for that invigorating minty flavor.

4. Squeeze the juice of one lime into the blender. Lime juice adds a zesty and refreshing kick.

5. If you desire added sweetness, add a tablespoon of honey. Adjust the amount based on your taste preference.

6. Include the Greek yogurt to create creaminess and boost the protein content.

7. Pour in your choice of coconut water (or your preferred liquid) to create the desired consistency. You can adjust the quantity to achieve your preferred thickness.

8. If you prefer an extra chill, add ice cubes to the blender.

9. Blend all the ingredients until you achieve a smooth, light green, and velvety texture.

10. Taste your Cucumber Mint Cooler and adjust the flavor if necessary. You can add more honey

for sweetness or more coconut water for a thinner consistency.

Serving Suggestion:
Pour your freshly blended Cucumber Mint Cooler into a chilled glass. Garnish with a sprig of fresh mint or a cucumber slice for an added visual appeal. This smoothie is ideal for sipping on a warm day, as a refreshing afternoon snack, or as a post-workout revitalizer. It's a reminder that staying hydrated and refreshed can be a delicious and invigorating experience.
The Cucumber Mint Cooler smoothie is like a sip of pure rejuvenation. Its blend of cucumber's coolness and mint's invigoration creates a harmonious and revitalizing experience. Make this smoothie a part of your hydration routine to enjoy the benefits of staying refreshed and invigorated while treating your taste buds to a delightful and cooling sensation. It's a testament to how simple ingredients can create a truly refreshing and nutritious beverage.

Raspberry Oatmeal Elixir

The Raspberry Oatmeal Elixir smoothie is a hearty and satisfying creation that combines the sweet-tartness of raspberries with the wholesome goodness of oats. This elixir is designed to not only tantalize your taste buds but also provide you with long-lasting energy and essential nutrients. It's the perfect choice for a fulfilling breakfast or a mid-day pick-me-up that keeps you fueled and focused.

Ingredients:

- 1 cup of fresh or frozen raspberries
- 1/2 cup of rolled oats
- 1/2 banana (frozen or fresh)
- 1/2 cup of Greek yogurt (or a dairy-free alternative)
- 1 tablespoon of honey (optional, for added sweetness)
- 1/2 cup of almond milk (or your preferred milk)

- A handful of ice cubes (optional)

Nutritional Benefits:

The Raspberry Oatmeal Elixir smoothie offers a range of health benefits:

- Raspberries: Raspberries are rich in antioxidants, fiber, and vitamins, particularly vitamin C, which supports immune health.

- Oats: Rolled oats provide a hearty source of fiber, which can help keep you feeling full and satisfied.

- Banana: Banana adds creaminess and natural sweetness along with potassium, an essential mineral for various bodily functions.

- Greek Yogurt: Greek yogurt contributes creaminess and an extra protein boost to promote satiety.

- Honey (Optional): Honey can enhance sweetness if desired, and it offers potential antibacterial and anti-inflammatory properties.

- Almond Milk: Unsweetened almond milk complements the flavors without adding unnecessary sugars.

Instructions:

1. Start by adding the fresh or frozen raspberries to your blender. Raspberries provide a delightful burst of color and flavor.

2. Include the rolled oats to infuse the smoothie with heartiness and fiber.

3. Add the frozen or fresh banana for creaminess and natural sweetness.

4. Spoon in the Greek yogurt for creaminess and an extra protein boost.

5. If you desire added sweetness, add a tablespoon of honey. Adjust the amount based on your taste preference.

6. Pour in your choice of almond milk (or your preferred milk) to create the desired consistency. You can adjust the quantity to achieve your preferred thickness.

7. If you prefer a colder, frostier smoothie, consider adding a handful of ice cubes.

8. Blend all the ingredients until you achieve a smooth, velvety texture. The result should be a vibrant, pinkish elixir that's as visually appealing as it is nutritious.

9. Taste your Raspberry Oatmeal Elixir and adjust the flavor if necessary. You can add more honey for sweetness or more almond milk for a thinner consistency.

Serving Suggestion:

Pour your freshly blended Raspberry Oatmeal Elixir into a tall glass. For an extra touch of elegance, garnish with a few fresh raspberries or a sprinkle of rolled oats. This smoothie is perfect for breakfast, as a mid-day energy booster, or as a pre-workout snack. It's a reminder that wholesome ingredients can create a delightful and nutritious elixir that fuels both body and soul.

The Raspberry Oatmeal Elixir smoothie is a testament to the satisfying power of oats and the vibrant appeal of raspberries. Its blend of hearty oats and juicy raspberries creates a wholesome and flavorful elixir that's perfect for starting your day with energy and nutrition. Incorporate this smoothie into your routine to enjoy the benefits of fiber, vitamins, and antioxidants while indulging in the delightful flavors of raspberries. It's a delicious reminder that a nutritious breakfast can be as enjoyable as it is nourishing.

Strawberry Spinach Surprise

Prepare to be pleasantly surprised by the Strawberry Spinach Surprise smoothie. This recipe beautifully marries the sweet juiciness of strawberries with the vibrant goodness of spinach, creating a concoction that's as visually appealing as it is delicious. Packed with vitamins, minerals, and antioxidants, this smoothie is the perfect choice for those looking to boost their nutrient intake while enjoying a burst of natural sweetness.

Ingredients:
- 1 cup of fresh strawberries, hulled and halved
- 1 cup of fresh spinach leaves
- 1/2 banana (frozen or fresh)
- 1/2 cup of Greek yogurt (or a dairy-free alternative)
- 1 tablespoon of honey (optional, for added sweetness)
- 1/2 cup of coconut water (or your preferred liquid)
- A handful of ice cubes (optional)

Nutritional Benefits:

The Strawberry Spinach Surprise smoothie offers a wealth of health benefits:

- Strawberries: Strawberries are rich in vitamin C, antioxidants, and dietary fiber, supporting immune health and digestion.

- Spinach: Spinach provides a host of vitamins and minerals, including vitamin K, folate, and iron, contributing to overall well-being.

- Banana: Banana adds creaminess, natural sweetness, and potassium for muscle function and blood pressure regulation.

- Greek Yogurt: Greek yogurt contributes creaminess and an extra protein boost to promote satiety.

- Honey (Optional): Honey can enhance sweetness if desired and may offer potential antibacterial and anti-inflammatory properties.

- Coconut Water: Coconut water complements the flavors without adding unnecessary sugars.

Instructions:

1. Begin by hulling and halving the fresh strawberries. This ensures a smooth blend.

2. Add the strawberries to your blender. Their vibrant red hue promises a delightful flavor burst.

3. Include the fresh spinach leaves for a nutritious and vibrant green addition.

4. Toss in the frozen or fresh banana for creaminess and natural sweetness.

5. Spoon in the Greek yogurt to add creaminess and an extra protein boost.

6. If you desire added sweetness, add a tablespoon of honey. Adjust the amount based on your taste preference.

7. Pour in your choice of coconut water (or your preferred liquid) to create the desired consistency. You can adjust the quantity to achieve your preferred thickness.

8. If you prefer a colder, frostier smoothie, consider adding a handful of ice cubes.

9. Blend all the ingredients until you achieve a smooth, visually striking blend that's both vibrant and nourishing.

10. Taste your Strawberry Spinach Surprise smoothie and adjust the flavor if necessary. You can add more honey for sweetness or more coconut water for a thinner consistency.

Serving Suggestion:

Pour your freshly blended Strawberry Spinach Surprise into a tall glass. For an added touch of elegance, garnish with a sliced strawberry or a spinach leaf. This smoothie is perfect for breakfast, as a mid-day nutrient booster, or as a refreshing post-workout recovery option. It's a reminder that nutrition can be a delightful and colorful journey.

The Strawberry Spinach Surprise smoothie is a delightful reminder of the beauty of vibrant ingredients. Its blend of sweet strawberries and nutrient-rich spinach creates a refreshing and visually stunning concoction that's as enjoyable as it is nourishing. Make this smoothie a part of your daily routine to enjoy the benefits of vitamins, minerals, and antioxidants while treating your taste buds to a naturally sweet surprise. It's proof that healthy choices can be both delicious and nutritious.

Avocado Avenger

Get ready to meet the "Avocado Avenger," a smoothie that not only delights your taste buds but also unleashes the nutritional power of avocados. Creamy, luscious, and satisfying, this green superhero is on a mission to provide you with essential nutrients and healthy fats while helping you achieve your weight loss goals. It's a delicious and creamy treat that combines the unique flavor of avocado with a touch of sweetness.

Ingredients:
- 1 ripe avocado, peeled and pitted
- 1/2 banana (frozen or fresh)
- 1/2 cup of Greek yogurt (or a dairy-free alternative)
- 1 tablespoon of honey (optional, for added sweetness)
- 1/2 cup of almond milk (or your preferred milk)
- A handful of ice cubes (optional)

Nutritional Benefits:

The "Avocado Avenger" smoothie offers a range of health benefits:

- Avocado: Avocado is a nutritional powerhouse, rich in heart-healthy monounsaturated fats, fiber, and various vitamins and minerals.

- Banana: Banana adds creaminess, natural sweetness, and potassium, which is essential for muscle function and maintaining proper blood pressure.

- Greek Yogurt: Greek yogurt contributes creaminess and an extra protein boost to promote satiety.

- Honey (Optional): Honey can enhance sweetness if desired and may offer potential antibacterial and anti-inflammatory properties.

- Almond Milk: Unsweetened almond milk complements the flavors without adding unnecessary sugars.

Instructions:

1. Begin by peeling and pitting the ripe avocado, ensuring you remove the pit.

2. Add the avocado flesh to your blender. Avocado is the star of this creamy show, bringing a rich, buttery texture to the mix.

3. Include the frozen or fresh banana to contribute creaminess and natural sweetness.

4. Spoon in the Greek yogurt to add creaminess and an extra protein boost.

5. If you desire added sweetness, add a tablespoon of honey. Adjust the amount based on your taste preference.

6. Pour in your choice of almond milk (or your preferred milk) to create the desired consistency. You can adjust the quantity to achieve your preferred thickness.

7. If you prefer a colder, more refreshing smoothie, consider adding a handful of ice cubes.

8. Blend all the ingredients until you achieve a smooth, creamy texture. The result should be a velvety, pale green creation that's both creamy and luscious.

9. Taste your Avocado Avenger smoothie and adjust the flavor if necessary. You can add more

honey for sweetness or more almond milk for a thinner consistency.

Serving Suggestion:

Pour your freshly blended Avocado Avenger into a chilled glass. This smoothie is so creamy and satisfying that it stands well on its own. However, you can also garnish it with a thin avocado slice or a drizzle of honey for an extra touch of elegance. Enjoy this smoothie for breakfast or as a filling snack to experience the full power of avocados.

The "Avocado Avenger" smoothie is a testament to the unique and creamy allure of avocados. Its blend of ripe avocado and other nutritious ingredients creates a smooth and satisfying concoction that's both creamy and delectable. Incorporate this smoothie into your daily routine to enjoy the benefits of healthy fats, fiber, and essential nutrients, all while indulging in a treat that's both nutritious and delightful. It's a reminder that achieving your weight loss goals can be as enjoyable as it is nourishing.

Orange Creamsicle Dream

Indulge in a nostalgic treat without the guilt with the "Orange Creamsicle Dream" smoothie. This delightful concoction captures the classic combination of sweet and tangy oranges with the lusciousness of a creamy creamsicle. It's a reminder that you can savor the flavors of childhood while nourishing your body with a nutritious and weight-loss-friendly option.

Ingredients:

- 2 large oranges, peeled and segmented
- 1/2 cup of Greek yogurt (or a dairy-free alternative)
- 1 tablespoon of honey (optional, for added sweetness)
- 1/2 cup of unsweetened almond milk (or your preferred milk)
- 1/2 teaspoon of pure vanilla extract
- A handful of ice cubes (optional)

Nutritional Benefits:

The "Orange Creamsicle Dream" smoothie offers a variety of health benefits:

- Oranges: Oranges are packed with vitamin C, antioxidants, and dietary fiber, supporting immune health and digestion.
- Greek Yogurt: Greek yogurt contributes creaminess and an extra protein boost to promote satiety.
- Honey (Optional): Honey can enhance sweetness if desired, and it may offer potential antibacterial and anti-inflammatory properties.
- Almond Milk: Unsweetened almond milk complements the flavors without adding unnecessary sugars.
- Vanilla Extract: Pure vanilla extract enhances the creamsicle flavor without added sugars.

Instructions:

1. Begin by peeling and segmenting the two large oranges. Removing the peel ensures a smoother blend.
2. Add the orange segments to your blender. Oranges provide a vibrant burst of sweet and tangy flavor.
3. Spoon in the Greek yogurt to add creaminess and a protein boost to the mix.

4. If you desire added sweetness, add a tablespoon of honey. Adjust the amount based on your taste preference.

5. Pour in your choice of unsweetened almond milk (or your preferred milk) to create the desired consistency. You can adjust the quantity to achieve your preferred thickness.

6. Add half a teaspoon of pure vanilla extract to enhance the creamsicle flavor.

7. If you prefer a colder, more refreshing smoothie, consider adding a handful of ice cubes.

8. Blend all the ingredients until you achieve a smooth, creamy, and vibrant orange texture.

9. Taste your Orange Creamsicle Dream smoothie and adjust the flavor if necessary. You can add more honey for sweetness or more almond milk for a thinner consistency.

Serving Suggestion:
Pour your freshly blended Orange Creamsicle Dream into a chilled glass. This smoothie is a creamy and flavorful treat that's perfect on its own. However, for a touch of nostalgia, you can

garnish it with a thin orange slice or a sprinkle of orange zest. Enjoy this smoothie for breakfast or as a refreshing dessert-like indulgence any time of day.

The "Orange Creamsicle Dream" smoothie is a delightful reminder of the classic combination of citrus and cream. Its blend of sweet and tangy oranges with the creamy allure of a creamsicle creates a smooth and satisfying concoction that's perfect for those moments when you're craving a nostalgic treat. Make this smoothie a part of your daily routine to enjoy the benefits of vitamin C, protein, and antioxidants while savoring the comforting flavors of an orange creamsicle. It's proof that nutritious choices can also be delicious and indulgent.

Chia Seed Cherry Charger

Get ready to charge up your day with the "Chia Seed Cherry Charger" smoothie. This vibrant blend combines the sweet and tart allure of cherries with the added goodness of chia seeds, creating a revitalizing concoction that's both delicious and nutritious. Packed with antioxidants, fiber, and essential nutrients, this smoothie is your ideal partner for an energy boost and weight loss journey.

Ingredients:

- 1 cup of fresh or frozen cherries, pitted

- 1 tablespoon of chia seeds

- 1/2 banana (frozen or fresh)

- 1/2 cup of Greek yogurt (or a dairy-free alternative)

- 1 tablespoon of honey (optional, for added sweetness)

- 1/2 cup of almond milk (or your preferred milk)

- A handful of ice cubes (optional)

Nutritional Benefits:

The "Chia Seed Cherry Charger" smoothie offers a range of health benefits:

- Cherries: Cherries are rich in antioxidants and vitamins, particularly vitamin C, which supports immune health.

- Chia Seeds: Chia seeds are a fantastic source of fiber, healthy fats, and protein, promoting feelings of fullness and supporting digestion.

- Banana: Banana adds creaminess, natural sweetness, and potassium for overall health.

- Greek Yogurt: Greek yogurt contributes creaminess and an extra protein boost to promote satiety.

- Honey (Optional): Honey can enhance sweetness if desired and may offer potential antibacterial and anti-inflammatory properties.

- Almond Milk: Unsweetened almond milk complements the flavors without adding unnecessary sugars.

Instructions:

1. Start by pitting the fresh cherries if they are not already pitted.

2. Add the pitted cherries to your blender. The vibrant color and sweet-tart flavor of cherries will be a highlight of your smoothie.

3. Sprinkle the chia seeds into the blender to add a dose of healthy fats, fiber, and protein.

4. Toss in the frozen or fresh banana for creaminess and natural sweetness.

5. Spoon in the Greek yogurt to create creaminess and boost the protein content.

6. If you desire added sweetness, add a tablespoon of honey. Adjust the amount based on your taste preference.

7. Pour in your choice of almond milk (or your preferred milk) to create the desired consistency. You can adjust the quantity to achieve your preferred thickness.

8. If you prefer a colder, frostier smoothie, consider adding a handful of ice cubes.

9. Blend all the ingredients until you achieve a smooth and velvety texture. The result should be a vibrant and inviting cherry concoction with a hint of chia texture.

10. Taste your Chia Seed Cherry Charger smoothie and adjust the flavor if necessary. You can add more honey for sweetness or more almond milk for a thinner consistency.

Serving Suggestion:

Pour your freshly blended Chia Seed Cherry Charger into a chilled glass. This smoothie is perfect for breakfast or as a pre-workout energy booster. For an extra touch of elegance, garnish with a few whole cherries or a sprinkle of chia seeds. It's a reminder that you can enjoy the sweet-tart flavors of cherries while giving your body the energy it needs to charge through the day.

The "Chia Seed Cherry Charger" smoothie is an energizing and satisfying blend that celebrates the natural sweetness of cherries and the power of chia seeds. Its combination of antioxidants,

fiber, and essential nutrients makes it an ideal
choice for those seeking an energy boost on their
weight loss journey. Incorporate this smoothie
into your daily routine to enjoy the benefits of
these nutritious ingredients while savoring the
delightful flavor of cherries. It's proof that
healthy choices can be both energizing and
delicious.

Peachy Keen Quencher

Quench your thirst and invigorate your taste buds with the "Peachy Keen Quencher" smoothie. This delightful concoction combines the luscious sweetness of ripe peaches with the hydrating freshness of coconut water. It's the perfect way to stay refreshed, keep your energy levels up, and support your weight loss journey with a burst of natural flavor and hydration.

Ingredients:

- 2 ripe peaches, peeled and pitted

- 1/2 cup of fresh pineapple chunks

- 1/2 cup of Greek yogurt (or a dairy-free alternative)

- 1/2 cup of coconut water

- 1 tablespoon of honey (optional, for added sweetness)

- A handful of ice cubes (optional)

Nutritional Benefits:

The "Peachy Keen Quencher" smoothie offers a variety of health benefits:

- Peaches: Peaches are rich in vitamins, particularly vitamin C, and dietary fiber, supporting immune health and digestion.

- Pineapple: Pineapple provides natural sweetness, along with vitamin C and enzymes that may aid digestion.

- Greek Yogurt: Greek yogurt contributes creaminess and an extra protein boost to promote satiety.

- Coconut Water: Coconut water is a natural hydrator, providing essential electrolytes without added sugars.

- Honey (Optional): Honey can enhance sweetness if desired, and it may offer potential antibacterial and anti-inflammatory properties.

Instructions:

1. Begin by peeling and pitting the ripe peaches. Removing the pits ensures a smoother blend.

2. Add the peeled and pitted peaches to your blender. The sweet and juicy flavor of peaches is a highlight of this quenching smoothie.

3. Toss in the fresh pineapple chunks for added sweetness and a tropical twist.

4. Include the Greek yogurt to create creaminess and an extra protein boost for satiety.

5. If you desire added sweetness, add a tablespoon of honey. Adjust the amount based on your taste preference.

6. Pour in the coconut water, which adds a natural and hydrating element to the mix.

7. If you prefer a colder, more refreshing smoothie, consider adding a handful of ice cubes.

8. Blend all the ingredients until you achieve a smooth, vibrant, and hydrating blend.

9. Taste your Peachy Keen Quencher smoothie and adjust the flavor if necessary. You can add more honey for sweetness or more coconut water for a thinner consistency.

Serving Suggestion:

Pour your freshly blended Peachy Keen Quencher into a tall glass. This smoothie is perfect for sipping on a warm day, as a refreshing afternoon pick-me-up, or as a post-workout revitalizer. For an extra touch of freshness, garnish with a slice of peach or a pineapple wedge. It's a reminder that staying hydrated can be a delicious and revitalizing experience.

The "Peachy Keen Quencher" smoothie is a celebration of the sweet and refreshing qualities of peaches, combined with the tropical appeal of pineapple and the hydrating power of coconut water. This concoction provides a burst of natural flavors and essential nutrients, making it the perfect choice for staying refreshed and hydrated during your weight loss journey. Incorporate this smoothie into your routine to enjoy the benefits of vitamins, hydration, and a delightful combination of flavors. It's proof that staying quenched can be as enjoyable as it is nourishing.